DAYS OF PANDEMIC

ANDREW ALDRED

chipmunkapublishing
the mental health publisher

Published by
Chipmunkapublishing
United Kingdom

http://www.chipmunkapublishing.com

ISBN   978-1-78382-5301

Dedication

"To my partner and best friend Jane".

Start Your Protest at Home

I saw the climate change protesters on TV today
Chaining themselves to car axles in London
But if they want to change the world for the better
I think they should sell their cars and get bicycles
And not go on foreign holidays, and if they do this
They will be doing their bit to change the world
And not pissing everyone off in the capital city

Dog Fouling

I saw a woman outside the house today
And her dog was ready to have a crap
She pulled it away rapidly when she saw me
And said she always poop-scooped and the shit on the pavement
Wasn't her dog's so I pulled her up
And said it was a constant problem
And if it didn't stop, I would get in touch with the council
So, the ball is in her court now
I'll wait and see what she and her doggie friends do!

Royalty

Prince Harry and Meghan Markle are on the news again
Promoting things that are dear to themselves and Princess Diana
And they do attract attention to some important things
Like the landmines that still exist all over Africa
The fact that conservation and creating a smaller carbon footprint
Is the key to humans and the planet surviving?
But Harry also puts his foot in it in some ways
It's alright for him and his wife to fly in a private jet
And he wants to fight a battle with the newspapers
Very probably because of how his mother was hounded by them
If I could give him some advice it would be
That he doesn't have to live a short and tragic life
And he doesn't need to make enemies of the people
That he will be looking to for support in the future
He's got a voice and he need to be responsible and use it well

ANDREW ALDRED

Vauxhall Astra

I've got a ten-year-old Vauxhall Astra now
It's the best car I've ever had
I'm trying to keep it in good repair
I bought a new door lining for it recently
And a new mirror for the driver's side
I fitted them myself
I've sprayed some bad paintwork
I'm keeping on top of things
I don't want the expense of a new car
This one doesn't leak oil
And I haven't crashed it yet!
I hope I can keep this car for a while

Avoiding the Off-License

I used to go to the off-license two or three nights a week
And they saw a middle-aged man buying beer
These women draw all sorts of conclusions
But I don't want to get involved with them
I've got a twelve-year relationship with the woman I love
I'm not easy and I'm not a "just for the night" type
I've got people that rely and me and I won't let them down
I'll be getting my beer somewhere else from now on

ANDREW ALDRED

I No Longer Suffer at Night

Since I turned fifty-three there's been a change in my life
I no longer wake up with a bloody arse
I haven't had piles for a long while
Who or whatever it is that has been bothering me for thirty years'?
Has moved on to somebody else
I'm free but in a poor state of health
I hope the powers that be have written me off
I don't know how I will be able to work again
The neighbours think that just because I can mow the lawn
And cut the hedge I should be working
They don't know how my illness has affected me
I don't know anyone, and I haven't got a clue where to start
Back into the world of employment again
And what would I really be fit for after this?

Old Age

Old age will get to us all if we live that long
I'm seeing my bones grow weaker and getting shorter of breath
Starting to become incontinent and salivate excessively
And I know I might have a hell of a long way to go
In this body that is beginning to fail me
You can face your demise kicking and screaming
Or you can have some dignity and go quietly
But you will never get the time back
Billy Connolly got is right when he said
"You've got to embrace it and get on with it"
Death is the common denominator and it will come to us all

ANDREW ALDRED

Disabled Comedienne

I saw her on Jonathan Ross this weekend
The comedienne with cerebral palsy
I think it would have been better if she had
Some sort of aid to help her speak fluently
She had some original jokes and was rude
Very self-effacing but she really had a go
And if people will pay to watch her
You've got to give her credit for trying to do something
But will she really be around in a few years?

DAYS OF PANDEMIC

Just Passing this Way

The planet has been around for a long time
And it wasn't always occupied by mankind
We've seen dinosaurs and the ice age
Come and pass before we existed
Global warming has been happening for a long time
And we overestimate our control over it
We may as well get on with living
And bear in mind one day we'll be extinct
Because the earth will no longer support us
It's time we stopped trying to play God
And realised we're just passing this way
And maybe God will take us back when we die

Underwater Cities

The sea is gradually swallowing the land up
As the ice caps melt and the water level rises
We're experiencing problems with flooding inland
And relocating our homes seems the only solution
People feel that global warming is all down to us
I say that it has been going on since time immemorial
But we are left with the problem of our territory shrinking
Maybe all that's left of us will be underwater cities?

Awkward

I don't want to have to bury my mum and dad
I can't face my relatives, they wouldn't understand
And I can't tell them anything about how I feel
I've just got to let everything pass quietly when the time comes
I understand myself and that's the important thing
Other people don't need to know anything
I'll deal with my problems and let the rest of them get on

So Tired

I get up late and try to get on with things
But by the afternoon I am tired again
It's a never-ending circle of fatigue
That I can't break out of
I wish I knew why I feel so tired
But I guess it wouldn't change a thing
And the best I can do is go to sleep

Change Isn't Always Good

What is so bad about Britain today?
Why do we want an independent Scotland?
Why do we want to get out of Europe?
If you're asking me, I don't bloody well know
I think we want to keep Britain as it is
I think we need to stay part of the European Union
And I think we ought to stop complaining
About people coming over because our country is better than theirs
Why can't we leave things as they are?
Why can't we look at the problem with homeless people?
And sort out our own country instead of looking at bigger issues?
Brexit has been a huge waste of time and resources
We need to stop being stupid and rocking the boat
Because we are the ones who will fall out
And that will be bad for everyone
Because I always had your best interests at heart

ANDREW ALDRED

Rainbow Poppies

The poppy is a symbol of remembrance
It doesn't consider what gender you are
Or what race, religion, colour or nationality
We are remembering people who died for our country
And if people of different sexuality want a rainbow poppy
They can have one, but I don't feel that will be necessary for me
I will be happy wearing a red poppy this year and every year
This represents my memories and those of the people I knew

DAYS OF PANDEMIC

Not Moving

She's been in the town centre for six months now
Summer has passed and winter is coming
And I'm wondering what the hell is wrong with her
That she won't accept help and get some accommodation
She never asks me for anything
I've got to guess she's alright
I knew her from ten years ago in mental hospital
I suppose she doesn't want to go back
Maybe it's more trouble than her life's worth
But a cold winter is coming, and I don't know if she'll survive

Genetic Engineering

Messing with genetics is very dangerous
You might get something you really don't want
It is a waste of resources and will not lead to a happy life
All these women over forty wanting a baby
And these gay couples who want a child
Should seriously consider being foster parents
Because there are enough children already there
Without putting genetically imperfect children
Into a world that is hard enough anyway
Genetic engineering is thoroughly wrong and abhorrent
And should be banned at every level
We need to make the best of what's already here

Milking It

She's coming back to Manchester
They're giving tickets away on the radio
But we won't be going
It's no longer two thousand and five
And the anthems feel so old
The tour smacks of keep me in my mansion
And send my kids to private school
She's overweight and getting past it
She reminds us too much of ourselves
Sorry Christina, but I guess you're an embarrassment
And we won't be going to see you this time

Birth Control

I don't understand these people who want a dozen children
When they only have the time to give to one or two
They don't go to work and drain the state's money
They haven't heard of contraceptives
I think there should be a law of two children per family
There are too many people in the world already
And we blame global warming on animals
We are animals and we are strangling the planet
There are more of us than anything else
We won't solve the world's problems by becoming vegetarian
Birth control is what is needed
Two children per family
Will sort out the world's problems

DAYS OF PANDEMIC

Into the Image

It seems if you want to be a successful rapper
All you do is have tattoos on your face
The music is all much the same
The lyrics are meaningless
Music used to be so memorable
But Post Malone and his crew are just so much blurb
It's more about the image than anything else
There's only one original song in the American top twenty
The other nineteen tracks might as well be the same song
They just feature different people in the videos
Where's the Rihanna's and the Lady Gaga's
The Beyoncé's, Snoop Dogg's and Eminem's
There's nobody to replace these people
Just a bunch of clones with no individuality and nothing to say

Everything to Everyone

I'm so bored of these celebrities
Who think they can be gay and father children?
Be transvestite, gay and straight at the same time
They're so big-headed and so ignorant
In their over-privileged ivory towers
Of the rest of us who are just trying to get on with our lives
You've got a choice of things
You can be transvestite, transsexual, gay, or straight
As a man or as a woman
And you will become one of these
Because eventually you will have to resort to something
You can't be everything to everyone
Be yourself and get on with it

Horrible Boss

I guess I'll always wonder why she was there
In her position of power, she used to abuse me
A thoroughly modern woman in every way
Career professional, single parent and probably lesbian
She hated her ex-husband who was in the army
And tried to take out her failed marriage on me
As I was called to see her one day in her office
I tried to explain to her that marriage is a two-way street
And that the breakdown of mine was not entirely my fault
But she reduced me to tears with her hatred
Of mentally ill people and ex-soldiers
If you hate mentally ill people, why work with them?
As a figure of considerable power and responsibility
Maybe you should be trying to help those under you
Or maybe you are on the wrong side of the fence
And you should be mentally ill, incarcerated and disempowered

ANDREW ALDRED

Waging War with Society

It's always a pity for those that cannot see the bigger picture
The outcasts in this world who have lost hope
But you need to somehow fit into the fabric of society
There is a pigeonhole for everyone and one for you
If you can't fit in where you are you can go up or down
You can always make things worse for yourself
If you are dissatisfied and want to strike out
You might as well be happy with what you have got
Or at least try to make things better for everyone
Because this will rub off on you and the rest of the world
Waging war with society has always been wrong and unproductive

Wallowing in Misery

If everyone was like you what a sad place the world would be
If things are bad, they can probably get worse
And you had better view your situation with a sense of humour
Because that is all that will get you through
The devil might care if nobody else does
It's too easy to get swallowed up by your own problems
There are billions of other people in the world
Some are better off than you and some worse
You need to get your problems in perspective
Wallowing in misery can kill you if your problems don't
Cheer up and get on with it and realise it won't last forever

Spent Force

I look back at my life and realise
I spent the best days of my life
With my ex-wife who is now my girlfriend
We made up for a lot of lost time
But now we're old and knackered
I can watch those girls on late night television
I could take somebody else if I wanted to
But it would never be as good
I see her every day of my life
We still look good together
But I've got to admit I'm past it now
I've had my best years and I'm a spent force

DAYS OF PANDEMIC

Greta Thunberg

Anyone and everyone are aware of climate change
But they have made Greta Thunberg some sort of figurehead for it
What is she saying and what solutions has she got?
She just wants to mouth off some load of childish crap
To anyone who will listen
Her parents should tell her to go to school
And think about her own future
Let the people in charge worry about the planet
Let the rest of us watch something else on TV
Do something useful instead of telling us what we already know

Asthma

They're telling me I've got asthma recently
I went to see the doctor and she gave me some tests
I told her I felt like I was drowning in bed
When I dreamt before waking up
My breathing is twenty per cent better with inhalers
It's just another health problem I don't need
I also smoke an e-cigarette continuously
Because I'm a bag of nerves with my mental illness
At least I have managed to give up smoking
But I'm growing older
And I might not manage my hedge in the garden
Because I'm too short of breath this year

Schizophrenic

Nobody wants the truth and it's in nobody's best interests
You must realise you're a pawn in a multi-dimensional game of
chess
You're involved with criminals and you're not totally innocent
Button your lip and get on with your life
Whatever you've done it's not that bad
Other people have far greater guilt and responsibility
You've got the fragments of a story but not the whole picture
It's just as well the world can say you're mentally ill
Because if that wasn't the case you could be dead

Gay Corporal

The dodgy moustache should have given him away
He's got a wife waiting for him at home
But younger men are all that really interests him
He's one of the best soldiers I have ever known
He can do a back flip in full kit
But the hardest thing he'll ever do
Is come out of the closet and admit he's gay

Just Desserts

We're all fighting a war out here
Everybody wants to hold someone else responsible
For their own grievances and problems
I've never crossed anyone who hasn't crossed me
And I really don't go looking for trouble
But I will pay for it like anyone else
And I hope I do that in this world
So, I can start the next one on a clean slate
Nobody I've ever met is totally innocent
And we will all get our just desserts

ANDREW ALDRED

Too Old to Play Soldiers

I know a man who is seventy-five years old
All he has ever lived for is the army
He reads books about special forces
His grandson has recently joined up
He's smart enough to see through some things
But he gets the wrong end of the stick with me
He wants to know about my service
But that's something I don't know so I can't declare it
I told him I was schizophrenic as soon as I met him
He has a place with the rest of them in the British Legion
But that's not my scene and I wouldn't fit in
I'm too old to play soldiers and at his age he should be too

Prophets of Doom

Donald Trump has been on the news again
Preaching about Socialism and American freedom
Citing Greta Thunberg as a prophet of doom
As the climate protesters mount another rally
But we should be aware they have a point
Donald Trump is also promising to plant a trillion trees
David Attenborough has prepared his witness statement
To the demise of humanity
I'm about as inland as it gets in Manchester
But there's flooding five miles away in Radcliffe
There's three times as many people inhabiting the earth
As there was when David Attenborough was born
Everyone can't get enough air and space
How are we ever going to put everything right?
The prophets of doom have something to say
And a message of goodwill by Donald Trump
Will do little to put everything right
We're choking on our own pollution and waste
But the world keeps turning on and on

Sex on TV

There's a programme called "Naked Attraction" on TV
And it's showing transgender people
Trying to build relationships with the rest of the world
I know we should acknowledge they exist
But this really isn't what I want to watch
Just like the girls with fake pubic hair
And the "Tattoo fixers" and "Take me out"
"Love Island", "Ex on the beach" and all the rest
It's all so different to my girlfriend and myself
We used to be married and now we're just partners
Life has pulled us far enough apart
But so many of these people really are grasping at straws
Relationships can be whatever you want
But people aren't content with normality any more
They want to bend things right out of shape
And put it on television for everyone to see

Lose Weight Well

There are a million different diets
And they all work on TV
Even if they don't in reality
They like to give you some hope
We all like watching TV
And half the world has too much to eat
If you consume a balanced diet
Without too many sugars, fats and carbohydrates
And eat a bit less than normal
And do as much exercise as possible
You will always lose weight
It can be a lifetime's work
You had better be determined
If you want to keep your figure

Pandemic

There's been ten thousand infected in China
We know this virus is contagious
There's been eight cases in the UK so far
The media is making a meal of it
There are isolation pods in every major hospital
And you just know everyone is going to get it
So, we might as well accept what is going to happen
It can't be contained, and we are all going to suffer

DAYS OF PANDEMIC

Philip Schofield

He's come out as gay at the age of fifty-seven
It's the bravest thing he's ever done
His adverts have suddenly disappeared on TV
He's married with children and has lived a lie
He said he was gay when he got married
So, this squeaky-clean character has skeletons in the closet
I never liked him very much
Maybe in a few years his past will catch up with him

Fame and Fragility

Fame and fragility don't go together
If you're in the public eye you had better be tough
Because the media will eat you like a pack of wolves
Harry and Meghan didn't last long
Princess Diana is long dead
Three suicides from Love Island in as many years
Celebrities frequently complaining about the press
Trolls and social media are the news
And everybody is so bloody vicious
If you're famous you've got to take the rough with the smooth
You will end up with a mixture of adulation and hatred
When asked whether her life had been worth the media frenzy
Amy Winehouse said on balance it wasn't
At least she made her mark, and what else would she have done?
If you don't thrive on aggravation
Keep out of the limelight and live a normal life

DAYS OF PANDEMIC

Find Somebody Else

I went to the off license to buy some beer
There was an Asian man at the counter
He called me darling and said something about paying the rent
I ignored him and walked out of the shop
Sorry son, but I can't do anything for you
Who the fuck do you people think you are?
Find somebody else or take a running jump at yourself
You run a supermarket, not a sex shop
And I'll be going back to Asda so I can avoid you

Ageist Policy

People are complaining because there are not enough over fifties
Being represented on TV in sexual situations
I'm more interested in getting on with being a grandparent
As far as my sex life goes, I've had it
It was good while it lasted and now, I'm knackered
And I can bet I represent a lot of people over fifty
Sexual scenes should be for the young and good-looking
My partner and I wouldn't want to get in front of a camera
With what we do for each other these days
If you've seen the trailer for "Bad Ass Grandma" on the adult
channel
It's enough to make you sick without seeing the film
Let the senior citizens get on with being retired
Look at "Last Tango in Halifax" and laugh
The lead actor is a gay man pretending to be straight
It's a ridiculous fantasy and that's what you get on TV
We should all be acting our age and not our shoe size
As someone over fifty I've no interest
In seeing people my age in sexual scenes on TV

DAYS OF PANDEMIC

Brutal

I watched the last episode of the Tyson Fury series today
And saw his remarkable rematch with Deontay Wilder
As Tyson Fury destroyed him viciously
In a way he will never recover from
Tyson Fury's father said it was unfinished business
And that he would bet his life on Tyson winning
How right he turned out to be
Tyson Fury is a very tough and durable man
And he sucked the life out of Deontay Wilder
Whilst not getting hurt or overly tired himself
He had to lose ten stone two years ago
Give up cocaine and alcohol and overcome mental illness
It is a remarkable lesson to us all
To never give up on what we are fighting for
He is a man with huge ambition and determination
But I think he has peaked, and this will be his greatest achievement

ANDREW ALDRED

Uncertain Times

We took her Mother's Day present to her today
She was isolated in a care home and we couldn't see her
We don't know whether we will be able to take our grandson home
To his mother in Manchester a week on Sunday
And we don't know whether we will be able to remain in contact
When the whole country is in lockdown because of the virus
We're isolating as a couple and doing our shopping
But we live separately and so much of our life is up in the air
In three months, we may be able to look back
See that we have got through alive and how far we have come
Will our parents still be alive, and will we?
It's hit Italy and Spain hard and it will come here
Time will see us through it but it's uncertain for everyone now

Bank Balance

It's difficult to know what's on Donald Trump's mind
When he makes his broadcast to the world at large
It seems he only cares about getting America back to work
And possible very little about the welfare of the people
When you know healthcare will come out of their pockets
Whilst they are all suffering from the virus
Bank balance is key and everything else is secondary
Mr Trump is a businessman through and through
With very little warmth and humanity in his soul
Boris Johnson's popularity has doubled during the virus
Whilst everybody keeps slating Donald Trump

ANDREW ALDRED

Stray Dogs

There's a couple of stray dogs in the area tonight
They are in the street barking because they are hungry
My pet rabbit stays in his cage
As I go out to check he's alright
I hope somebody telephones the dog catcher
And gets these strays impounded before they do any damage

Glory Holes

You can see the adverts for TVX 40 plus
Full of sluts falling to pieces in front of us
While they strut their stuff with two sexual partners
Or with their gay girlfriend
I watch for a while before I turn it off
And I begin to realise I don't understand these people
Are they looking for a relationship in a sea of sex?
It's difficult to have friends when everything is a sexual trade-off
Your glory hole should probable be something you shit out of
You see these people once or twice and it gets so boring

Barren Trees

I have two fruit trees in my garden
Neither have never bore any fruit
There's a pear tree for me and an apple tree for her
The pear tree is slender, and the apple tree is stunted
She grew the apple tree from a seed
And I rescued the pear tree from her mother's garden
Where it had been growing in a dustbin
They are symbolic of a couple who never had a baby
We wouldn't have been able to bring up a child
We were too old and had too many bad habits
I had a vasectomy and now she's going through menopause
Like our trees we live on. If only things had been different.

DAYS OF PANDEMIC

Self-isolation

Sometimes living in two separate houses is not a good idea
Like when the world is struck down by a bloody virus
You separate to look after your houses
And then there's my pet rabbit to be fed
We skype each other twice every day
And have frequent phone calls, I take her a meal
When I cook something in the slow cooker
I do shopping, we get deliveries when we can
We both have chronic health problems, but we are getting on
She's got stents in her heart and myalgia in her legs
I suffer from asthma and have had cancer and a heart blockage
But we have received no letter from the authorities
So, we will survive the best way we can
And hope we can live out the next few months

ANDREW ALDRED

Never be the same

The airlines have collapsed
It is a few degrees colder
And the air quality is already better
Since there are less cars on the road
We've all been choking on our pollution
For far too long now
There is a mass-culling of humans
But it might sort out the world's problems
And leave a better world for those left
Teach us to care about our planet
And not squander our lives
In a frenzied orgasm of activity
To love each other and our surroundings

A Different Kind of Hero

A lot of them are young and freshly trained
With some who have come back to the profession
Many of them have never raised a fist in anger
Let alone fire a bullet from a gun
But they are the new breed of hero
Frontline medical workers and supermarket staff
Engineers building the country's much needed equipment
To fight the deadly virus invading our country
Some might say it is worse for the military
But these people are from all walks of life
And just as worthy as any soldier ever was

ANDREW ALDRED

Hold on to Love

We hold on to our love the best way we can
With frequent telephone calls and skype messaging
I bring her shopping and food I have cooked
Try to talk her round when she is depressed
And she always answers the phone when I call
We need to hold on to our love the best way we can
And not be beaten by this bloody pandemic